DR. BARBARA'S MUCUS CLEANSE JUICING RECIPES

Discover Dr.Barbara's transformative mucus cleanse: obtain vibrant health and naturalhealing through full-body cleanse and detox

Ben Hans

Table of Contents

COPYRIGHT © 2023

CHAPTER ONE

Understanding Mucus: Exploring its Role in the Body

Mucus is a viscous, slimy substance produced by mucous membranes found in various parts of the body, including the respiratory, digestive, and reproductive systems. While it's often associated with discomfort when someone has a cold or flu, mucus actually serves several vital functions in the body. In this comprehensive exploration, we'll delve into the multifaceted role of mucus, its composition, production, and its significance in maintaining overall health and well-being.

Composition of Mucus

Mucus is primarily composed of water, glycoproteins, salts, enzymes, and antimicrobial substances. The glycoproteins, particularly mucins, are the key components responsible for its gel-like consistency. Mucins contain long carbohydrate chains called glycans, which provide mucus with its characteristic stickiness and lubricating properties. These glycans also facilitate the trapping and clearance of foreign particles, such as bacteria and viruses.

In addition to mucins, mucus contains various enzymes that play crucial roles in protecting the body from pathogens and aiding in digestion. Lysozyme, for example, has antimicrobial properties and helps break down bacterial cell walls. Other enzymes, such as amylase and lipase, assist in the digestion of carbohydrates and fats, respectively.

Functions of Mucus

1. **Protection**: One of the primary functions of mucus is to protect the body's mucous membranes from damage and infection. Mucus acts as a physical barrier, trapping foreign particles, pathogens, and toxins before they can penetrate deeper into tissues. This helps prevent infections and reduces the risk of inflammation and tissue damage.

2. **Lubrication**: Mucus serves as a lubricant in various physiological processes, such as swallowing, digestion, and reproductive activities. In the respiratory system, mucus keeps the airways moist and facilitates the movement of air into the lungs. In the digestive tract, mucus lubricates food particles, easing their passage through the esophagus and intestines.

3. **Immune Defense**: Mucus contains antimicrobial substances, including antibodies, enzymes, and proteins, which help neutralize pathogens and boost the body's immune response. These components act as the first line of defense against invading microorganisms, preventing infections and reducing the severity of illnesses.

4. **Moisture Regulation**: Mucus plays a crucial role in maintaining the moisture balance in various parts of the body, particularly in the respiratory and digestive systems. By keeping the mucous membranes moist, mucus helps prevent dryness, irritation, and discomfort, especially in environments with low humidity.

5. **Waste Removal**: Mucus also aids in the removal of waste products and toxins from the body. In the respiratory system, cilia—hair-like structures lining the airways—beat in coordinated waves, pushing mucus and trapped particles upward towards the throat, where they can be expelled through coughing or swallowing. Similarly, in the digestive tract, mucus helps move waste materials along the intestines for elimination.

Production of Mucus

Mucus is produced by specialized cells called goblet cells, which are scattered throughout the mucous membranes lining the respiratory, digestive, and reproductive tracts. These cells secrete mucus in response to various stimuli, such as irritation, inflammation, or the presence of pathogens. The production and composition of mucus can be influenced by factors such as hormonal changes, hydration status, and environmental conditions.

Once produced, mucus undergoes constant turnover, with old mucus being continuously cleared away and replaced by newly synthesized mucus. This turnover process helps maintain the integrity of the mucous membranes and ensures optimal functioning of the mucus layer.

Role of Mucus in Disease

While mucus plays a crucial role in protecting the body from infections and maintaining overall health, abnormalities in mucus production or composition can contribute to various diseases and health conditions. For example:

- **Respiratory Conditions**: Excessive mucus production or thickening of mucus can occur in respiratory conditions such as asthma, chronic bronchitis, and cystic fibrosis. This can lead to airway obstruction, breathing difficulties, and an increased risk of respiratory infections.

- **Gastrointestinal Disorders**: Inflammatory bowel diseases (IBD) such as Crohn's disease and ulcerative colitis are characterized by inflammation of the digestive tract, which can disrupt mucus production and secretion. This can impair the protective function of mucus, leading to tissue damage and gastrointestinal symptoms.

- **Reproductive Health**: Changes in cervical mucus consistency and production can affect fertility and reproductive health in women. Abnormalities in cervical mucus secretion may interfere with sperm transport and fertilization, leading to difficulties in conceiving.

Conclusion

In conclusion, mucus plays a diverse and essential role in maintaining the health and functioning of the body. From protecting mucous membranes to aiding in digestion and immune defense, mucus serves as a versatile biological substance with multifaceted functions. Understanding the composition, production, and significance of mucus provides valuable insights into its role in health and disease, highlighting the importance of maintaining mucus homeostasis for overall well-being.

CHAPTER TWO

The Benefits of Herbal Cleansing: A Comprehensive Overview

Herbal cleansing, also known as herbal detoxification or herbal cleansing therapy, is a holistic approach to wellness that involves using herbs and natural remedies to eliminate toxins from the body, support organ function, and promote overall health. This comprehensive overview will delve into the various benefits of herbal cleansing, including its effects on detoxification, digestion, immunity, and general well-being.

Detoxification

One of the primary benefits of herbal cleansing is its ability to support the body's natural detoxification processes. The human body is constantly exposed to toxins from various sources, including environmental pollutants, processed foods, medications, and stress. Over time, these toxins can accumulate in the body and impair organ function, leading to fatigue, digestive issues, skin problems, and other health problems.

Herbal cleansing therapies typically involve the use of herbs with detoxifying properties, such as dandelion root, burdock root, milk thistle, and turmeric. These herbs contain compounds that help stimulate the liver, kidneys, and lymphatic system, enhancing the elimination of toxins from the body. By supporting the body's detoxification pathways, herbal cleansing can help improve energy levels, mental clarity, and overall vitality.

Digestive Health

Another significant benefit of herbal cleansing is its positive impact on digestive health. The digestive system plays a crucial role in nutrient absorption, waste elimination, and immune function. Poor digestion can lead to a range of health issues, including bloating, gas, constipation, diarrhea, and inflammation.

Many herbal cleansing protocols include herbs that support digestive function, such as ginger, peppermint, fennel, and licorice root. These herbs have carminative, anti-inflammatory, and antimicrobial properties, which help soothe the digestive tract, relieve gastrointestinal discomfort, and promote healthy bowel movements. By improving digestion, herbal cleansing can enhance nutrient absorption, reduce bloating and gas, and support overall gut health.

Immune Support

Herbal cleansing can also provide immune support by strengthening the body's natural defenses against infections and illness. The immune system is responsible for identifying and neutralizing pathogens, such as bacteria, viruses, and fungi, to prevent infection and maintain health.

Certain herbs used in herbal cleansing, such as echinacea, elderberry, astragalus, and garlic, have immune-boosting properties that can help enhance immune function and reduce the risk of infections. These herbs contain bioactive compounds, such as flavonoids, polysaccharides, and alkaloids, which stimulate immune cells, increase antibody production, and exert antiviral and antibacterial effects. By supporting immune function, herbal cleansing can help the body resist infections and recover more quickly from illness.

Stress Reduction

Chronic stress can have a detrimental effect on physical and mental health, contributing to a range of conditions, including anxiety, depression, cardiovascular disease, and immune dysfunction. Herbal cleansing therapies often incorporate adaptogenic herbs, such as ashwagandha, holy basil, rhodiola, and Siberian ginseng, which help the body adapt to stress and promote relaxation.

Adaptogens are a class of herbs that help regulate the body's stress response by modulating the production of stress hormones, such as cortisol and adrenaline. These herbs have been used for centuries in traditional medicine systems, such as Ayurveda and Traditional Chinese Medicine, to promote resilience, vitality, and longevity. By supporting the body's ability to cope with stress, herbal cleansing can help reduce anxiety, improve mood, and enhance overall well-being.

Conclusion

In conclusion, herbal cleansing offers a wide range of benefits for detoxification, digestion, immunity, and stress reduction. By using herbs and natural remedies to support the body's innate healing mechanisms, herbal cleansing can help improve energy levels, promote digestive health, boost immune function, and reduce the negative effects of chronic stress. Incorporating herbal cleansing into a healthy lifestyle regimen can be an effective way to optimize health and vitality naturally.

CHAPTER THREE

Getting Started: Preparing for Your Mucus Cleanse Journey

Embarking on a mucus cleanse journey can be a transformative experience for your health and well-being. Whether you're seeking relief from respiratory issues, digestive discomfort, or simply aiming to optimize your overall vitality, a mucus cleanse can help you reset your body and restore balance. However, proper preparation is essential to ensure a safe and effective cleanse. In this guide, we'll explore the key steps to getting started on your mucus cleanse journey.

1. Set Clear Intentions

Before beginning your mucus cleanse, take some time to reflect on your reasons for undertaking this journey. What specific health goals do you hope to achieve? Are you seeking relief from respiratory symptoms, digestive issues, or general detoxification? Setting clear intentions will help you stay focused and motivated throughout the cleanse process.

2. Educate Yourself

Understanding the principles and practices of mucus cleansing is crucial for success. Take the time to research reputable sources, books, and articles on the topic to gain insights into how mucus affects your body and the most effective strategies for cleansing.

Familiarize yourself with different herbs, dietary protocols, and lifestyle practices that support mucus elimination and overall health.

3. Consult with a Healthcare Professional

Before starting any cleanse or detox program, it's essential to consult with a qualified healthcare professional, especially if you have any underlying health conditions or are taking medications. A healthcare provider can help assess your individual health status, provide personalized recommendations, and ensure that a mucus cleanse is safe and appropriate for you.

4. Assess Your Current Lifestyle

Take a close look at your current lifestyle habits, including diet, hydration, exercise, sleep, and stress management. Are there any areas where you can make improvements to support your cleanse journey? Consider reducing or eliminating processed foods, sugar, alcohol, and caffeine, which can contribute to mucus production and inflammation in the body. Aim to incorporate more whole, nutrient-dense foods, hydrating beverages, and stress-reducing activities into your daily routine.

5. Plan Your Cleanse Protocol

Once you've gathered information and consulted with a healthcare professional, it's time to design your mucus cleanse protocol. This may include a combination of dietary changes, herbal supplements, hydration strategies, and lifestyle practices tailored to your individual needs and goals. Some common components of a mucus cleanse protocol include:

- **Dietary Modifications**: Focus on consuming whole, plant-based foods rich in fiber, antioxidants, and essential nutrients. Incorporate plenty of fruits, vegetables, leafy greens, whole grains, legumes, nuts, and seeds into your meals. Avoid or minimize processed foods, dairy products, gluten, and inflammatory oils.

- **Hydration**: Drink plenty of water throughout the day to help thin mucus and facilitate its elimination from the body. Herbal teas, such as peppermint, ginger, and licorice root, can also support hydration and mucus clearance.

- **Herbal Supplements**: Consider incorporating herbal remedies known for their mucus-clearing and immune-supportive properties, such as marshmallow root, fenugreek, mullein, and elderberry. These herbs can be taken in various forms, including teas, tinctures, capsules, or powders.

- **Breathing Exercises**: Practice deep breathing exercises, such as diaphragmatic breathing or pranayama, to improve lung function, oxygenation, and mucus clearance in the respiratory tract.

- **Stress Management**: Engage in stress-reducing activities such as meditation, yoga, tai chi, or nature walks to promote relaxation, reduce cortisol levels, and support overall well-being.

6. Gather Supplies

Before you begin your mucus cleanse, gather all the supplies you'll need to support your journey. This may include herbal supplements, herbal teas, fresh produce, hydration tools (such as a water bottle or herbal infuser), and any other items specific to your cleanse protocol. Having everything prepared in advance will make it easier to stick to your plan and avoid last-minute obstacles.

7. Set Realistic Expectations

Keep in mind that mucus cleansing is not a quick fix or a one-size-fits-all solution. It's a gradual process that requires patience, consistency, and commitment. Be realistic about your expectations and understand that results may vary depending on individual factors such as health status, dietary habits, and lifestyle choices. Focus on the journey rather than the destination, and celebrate small victories along the way.

8. Stay Flexible and Listen to Your Body

As you embark on your mucus cleanse journey, listen to your body's signals and adjust your approach accordingly. Pay attention to how you feel physically, mentally, and emotionally throughout the cleanse process. If certain foods or practices don't agree with you, don't hesitate to make modifications or seek guidance from a healthcare professional. Remember that self-care and self-compassion are essential components of any healing journey.

By following these steps and preparing thoughtfully for your mucus cleanse journey, you'll set yourself up for success and maximize the benefits of this transformative experience. Embrace the opportunity to nourish your body, clear away toxins, and cultivate vibrant health from the inside out.

CHAPTER FOUR

Essential Juicing Tools and Ingredients

Juicing is a popular method for extracting nutrients from fruits, vegetables, and herbs, providing a convenient way to boost your intake of vitamins, minerals, and antioxidants. To create delicious and nutritious juices at home, you'll need a few essential tools and a variety of fresh ingredients. In this guide, we'll explore the must-have juicing tools and ingredients to help you get started on your juicing journey.

Essential Juicing Tools:

1. **Juicer**: The most essential tool for juicing is a high-quality juicer. There are two main types of juicers: centrifugal and masticating. Centrifugal juicers work by shredding fruits and vegetables with a fast-spinning blade, while masticating juicers use a slower, crushing action to extract juice. Masticating juicers are generally preferred for their ability to extract more juice and preserve nutrients, although centrifugal juicers are often more affordable and convenient for beginners.

2. **Cutting Board and Knife**: A sturdy cutting board and a sharp knife are essential for preparing fruits and vegetables for juicing. Choose a cutting board made of food-safe materials, such as wood or plastic, and opt for a knife with a

comfortable grip and a sharp blade for easy slicing and chopping.

3. **Juice Collection Container**: You'll need a container to collect the fresh juice as it's extracted from the fruits and vegetables. Many juicers come with built-in juice collection containers, but you can also use a pitcher, glass jar, or bowl to collect the juice.

4. **Strainer or Nut Milk Bag**: Depending on your juicer type and personal preference, you may need a strainer or nut milk bag to remove pulp and fiber from the juice. This can help create a smoother, more refined juice texture, especially if you prefer a pulp-free consistency.

5. **Cleaning Brush**: Proper cleaning is essential for maintaining your juicer and ensuring optimal performance. A cleaning brush specifically designed for juicers can help remove pulp and residue from hard-to-reach areas, making cleanup quick and easy.

6. **Storage Containers**: If you plan to make large batches of juice to enjoy throughout the day, consider investing in airtight storage containers or glass bottles for storing your fresh juice in the refrigerator. This will help preserve the freshness and flavor of the juice for longer periods.

Essential Juicing Ingredients:

1. **Leafy Greens**: Leafy greens such as kale, spinach, Swiss chard, and collard greens are nutrient powerhouses packed with vitamins, minerals, and antioxidants. They add vibrant color and a refreshing flavor to juices while providing essential nutrients for overall health and vitality.

2. **Fruits**: Choose a variety of ripe, fresh fruits to add sweetness and flavor to your juices. Popular options include apples, oranges, berries, pineapple, grapes, and citrus fruits such as lemons and limes. Experiment with different fruit combinations to create delicious and satisfying juice blends.

3. **Vegetables**: In addition to leafy greens, incorporate a variety of vegetables into your juices for added nutrition and flavor. Carrots, cucumbers, beets, celery, bell peppers, and ginger are excellent choices for juicing, providing a rich source of vitamins, minerals, and antioxidants.

4. **Herbs and Spices**: Fresh herbs and spices can elevate the flavor profile of your juices and provide additional health benefits. Add herbs such as parsley, cilantro, mint, or basil to your juice blends for a burst of freshness and aroma. Spices like turmeric, ginger, and cinnamon can add warmth and depth of flavor while offering anti-inflammatory and antioxidant properties.

5. **Citrus**: Citrus fruits such as lemons, limes, oranges, and grapefruits are popular ingredients for juicing due to their

bright, tangy flavor and high vitamin C content. Citrus fruits also contain bioactive compounds such as flavonoids and limonoids, which have antioxidant and immune-boosting properties.

6. **Root Vegetables**: Root vegetables like carrots, beets, and sweet potatoes are excellent choices for juicing, providing a natural sweetness and vibrant color to your juice blends. These vegetables are rich in vitamins, minerals, and antioxidants, making them valuable additions to your juicing repertoire.

7. **Superfoods**: Consider incorporating superfoods such as spirulina, wheatgrass, chlorella, and moringa into your juice blends for an extra nutritional boost. These nutrient-dense ingredients are rich in vitamins, minerals, amino acids, and antioxidants, providing potent health benefits and supporting overall well-being.

By stocking up on these essential juicing tools and ingredients, you'll be well-equipped to create delicious, nutrient-packed juices at home. Experiment with different flavor combinations, explore new ingredients, and enjoy the countless health benefits of juicing as you embark on your juicing journey.

CHAPTER FIVE

Morning Energizers: Revitalize with Refreshing Herbal Juices

Starting your day with a refreshing herbal juice can be a fantastic way to revitalize your body, boost your energy levels, and nourish your cells with essential nutrients. Herbal juices are not only delicious but also offer a wide range of health benefits, from supporting digestion to enhancing immune function. In this guide, we'll explore some invigorating herbal juice recipes designed to kickstart your morning and energize your day.

1. Green Goddess Juice:

Ingredients:

- 2 cups spinach leaves

- 1 cucumber

- 1 green apple

- 1/2 lemon (peeled)

- 1-inch piece of ginger (peeled)

- Handful of fresh mint leaves

Instructions:

1. Wash the spinach leaves, cucumber, apple, lemon, and ginger thoroughly.

2. Cut the cucumber and apple into chunks, removing any seeds or stems.

3. Peel the lemon and ginger.

4. Juice all the ingredients together, starting with the spinach leaves and alternating with the cucumber, apple, lemon, ginger, and mint leaves.

5. Stir the juice well and serve immediately over ice, if desired.

2. Citrus Sunshine Juice:

Ingredients:

- 2 oranges (peeled)

- 2 carrots

- 1 lemon (peeled)

- 1-inch piece of turmeric (peeled)

- 1-inch piece of ginger (peeled)

Instructions:

1. Wash the oranges, carrots, lemon, turmeric, and ginger.

2. Cut the oranges and lemon into quarters.

3. Peel the turmeric and ginger.

4. Juice all the ingredients together, starting with the oranges and alternating with the carrots, lemon, turmeric, and ginger.

5. Stir the juice well and pour into glasses.

3. Tropical Turmeric Twist:

Ingredients:

- 1 cup pineapple chunks

- 1 mango (peeled and pitted)

- 1 orange (peeled)

- 1-inch piece of turmeric (peeled)

- Handful of fresh cilantro leaves

Instructions:

1. Wash the mango, orange, turmeric, and cilantro leaves.

2. Cut the mango into chunks, discarding the pit.

3. Peel the orange and turmeric.

4. Juice all the ingredients together, starting with the pineapple chunks and alternating with the mango, orange, turmeric, and cilantro leaves.

5. Stir the juice well and serve immediately.

4. Ginger Zinger Juice:

Ingredients:

- 3 carrots

- 1 apple

- 1-inch piece of ginger (peeled)

- 1/2 lemon (peeled)

- Handful of fresh parsley leaves

Instructions:

1. Wash the carrots, apple, ginger, lemon, and parsley leaves.

2. Cut the carrots and apple into chunks, removing any seeds or stems.

3. Peel the ginger and lemon.

4. Juice all the ingredients together, starting with the carrots and alternating with the apple, ginger, lemon, and parsley leaves.

5. Stir the juice well and pour into glasses.

5. Cleansing Celery Cooler:

Ingredients:

- 4 celery stalks

- 1 cucumber

- 1 green apple

- 1/2 lemon (peeled)

- Handful of fresh cilantro leaves

Instructions:

1. Wash the celery stalks, cucumber, apple, lemon, and cilantro leaves.

2. Cut the cucumber and apple into chunks, removing any seeds or stems.

3. Peel the lemon.

4. Juice all the ingredients together, starting with the celery stalks and alternating with the cucumber, apple, lemon, and cilantro leaves.

5. Stir the juice well and serve over ice, if desired.

Tips for Enjoying Herbal Juices:

- Use organic ingredients whenever possible to minimize exposure to pesticides and chemicals.

- Experiment with different combinations of herbs, fruits, and vegetables to create your own unique juice blends.

- Drink your herbal juice immediately after juicing to maximize freshness and nutrient content.

- If you prefer a smoother juice texture, strain the juice through a fine mesh sieve or nut milk bag to remove pulp and fiber.

- Enjoy your herbal juice as part of a balanced breakfast or snack to fuel your body and promote optimal health and vitality.

By incorporating these invigorating herbal juice recipes into your morning routine, you can start your day on a refreshing and energizing note, supporting your overall health and well-being. Cheers to vibrant mornings and revitalized days with herbal juices!

CHAPTER SIX

Midday Rejuvenation: Nourish and Detoxify with Herbal Blends

As the day progresses, it's common to experience a dip in energy and concentration. Midday is the perfect time to recharge and refocus with a nourishing and detoxifying herbal blend. Herbal blends offer a convenient and effective way to replenish essential nutrients, support detoxification, and promote overall well-being. In this guide, we'll explore some rejuvenating herbal blends to help you power through the day feeling refreshed and revitalized.

1. Detoxifying Green Elixir:

Ingredients:

- 1 cup spinach leaves

- 1/2 cucumber

- 1 green apple

- 1/2 lemon (peeled)

- 1-inch piece of ginger (peeled)

- 1 tablespoon fresh parsley leaves

- 1 tablespoon fresh cilantro leaves

- 1 teaspoon spirulina powder

Instructions:

1. Wash the spinach leaves, cucumber, apple, lemon, ginger, parsley, and cilantro.

2. Cut the cucumber and apple into chunks, removing any seeds or stems.

3. Peel the lemon and ginger.

4. Juice all the ingredients together, starting with the spinach leaves and alternating with the cucumber, apple, lemon, ginger, parsley, and cilantro.

5. Stir in the spirulina powder until well combined.

6. Pour the elixir into a glass and enjoy immediately.

2. Refreshing Citrus Cleanse:

Ingredients:

- 2 oranges (peeled)

- 1 grapefruit (peeled)

- 1 lemon (peeled)

- 1-inch piece of turmeric (peeled)

- 1-inch piece of ginger (peeled)

- 1 tablespoon fresh mint leaves

- 1 teaspoon chlorella powder

Instructions:

1. Wash the oranges, grapefruit, lemon, turmeric, ginger, and mint leaves.

2. Cut the oranges, grapefruit, and lemon into quarters.

3. Peel the turmeric and ginger.

4. Juice all the ingredients together, starting with the oranges and alternating with the grapefruit, lemon, turmeric, ginger, and mint leaves.

5. Stir in the chlorella powder until well combined.

6. Pour the cleanse into a glass and enjoy immediately.

3. Berry Burst Antioxidant Blend:

Ingredients:

- 1 cup mixed berries (such as strawberries, blueberries, raspberries)
- 1/2 cup spinach leaves
- 1/2 cucumber
- 1 green apple
- 1/2 lemon (peeled)

- 1-inch piece of ginger (peeled)

- 1 tablespoon fresh basil leaves

- 1 teaspoon acai powder

Instructions:

1. Wash the berries, spinach leaves, cucumber, apple, lemon, ginger, and basil leaves.

2. Cut the cucumber and apple into chunks, removing any seeds or stems.

3. Peel the lemon and ginger.

4. Juice all the ingredients together, starting with the berries and alternating with the spinach leaves, cucumber, apple, lemon, ginger, and basil leaves.

5. Stir in the acai powder until well combined.

6. Pour the blend into a glass and enjoy immediately.

4. Tropical Turmeric Tonic:

Ingredients:

- 1 cup pineapple chunks

- 1 mango (peeled and pitted)

- 1 orange (peeled)

- 1-inch piece of turmeric (peeled)

- 1-inch piece of ginger (peeled)

- 1 tablespoon fresh cilantro leaves

- 1 teaspoon turmeric powder

Instructions:

1. Wash the mango, orange, turmeric, ginger, and cilantro leaves.

2. Cut the mango into chunks, discarding the pit.

3. Peel the orange, turmeric, and ginger.

4. Juice all the ingredients together, starting with the pineapple chunks and alternating with the mango, orange, turmeric, ginger, and cilantro leaves.

5. Stir in the turmeric powder until well combined.

6. Pour the tonic into a glass and enjoy immediately.

Tips for Enjoying Herbal Blends:

- Use organic ingredients whenever possible to minimize exposure to pesticides and chemicals.

- Experiment with different combinations of fruits, vegetables, and herbs to create your own unique herbal blends.

- Customize your blends by adding superfood powders such as spirulina, chlorella, acai, or turmeric for an extra nutritional boost.

- Enjoy your herbal blends as a midday pick-me-up or as a refreshing accompaniment to your lunch.

- Drink your herbal blends immediately after juicing to maximize freshness and nutrient content.

By incorporating these nourishing and detoxifying herbal blends into your midday routine, you can rejuvenate your body and mind, supporting your overall health and vitality. Cheers to vibrant midday moments with herbal goodness!

CHAPTER SEVEN

Afternoon Boosters: Sustain Energy Levels with Herbal Elixirs

As the afternoon slump sets in, it's essential to find ways to sustain your energy levels and stay focused and alert. Herbal elixirs offer a natural and rejuvenating way to boost your energy, support mental clarity, and enhance overall well-being. In this guide, we'll explore some invigorating herbal elixir recipes designed to provide sustained energy and vitality throughout the afternoon.

1. Energizing Matcha Latte:

Ingredients:

- 1 teaspoon matcha powder

- 1 cup unsweetened almond milk (or milk of choice)

- 1 teaspoon honey or maple syrup (optional)

- 1/2 teaspoon vanilla extract

- Pinch of cinnamon

Instructions:

1. In a small saucepan, heat the almond milk over medium heat until warm but not boiling.

2. In a mug, whisk together the matcha powder, honey or maple syrup (if using), vanilla extract, and cinnamon until smooth.

3. Slowly pour the warm almond milk into the matcha mixture, stirring continuously until well combined.

4. Froth the latte using a milk frother or immersion blender until foamy.

5. Serve the matcha latte immediately and enjoy the sustained energy boost.

2. Adaptogenic Ashwagandha Elixir:

Ingredients:

- 1 teaspoon ashwagandha powder

- 1 cup unsweetened coconut milk (or milk of choice)

- 1 teaspoon honey or maple syrup (optional)

- 1/2 teaspoon ground cardamom

- Pinch of nutmeg

Instructions:

1. In a small saucepan, heat the coconut milk over medium heat until warm but not boiling.

2. In a mug, whisk together the ashwagandha powder, honey or maple syrup (if using), ground cardamom, and nutmeg until well combined.

3. Slowly pour the warm coconut milk into the ashwagandha mixture, stirring continuously until smooth.

4. Sprinkle a pinch of ground cinnamon on top for extra flavor, if desired.

5. Serve the ashwagandha elixir immediately and savor the soothing and energizing benefits.

3. Brain-Boosting Ginseng Tonic:

Ingredients:

- 1 teaspoon ginseng powder

- 1 cup brewed green tea, cooled

- 1 tablespoon fresh lemon juice

- 1 teaspoon honey or maple syrup (optional)

- Ice cubes

Instructions:

1. In a glass, combine the ginseng powder, brewed green tea, fresh lemon juice, and honey or maple syrup (if using).

2. Stir the tonic until the ingredients are well mixed.

3. Add ice cubes to the glass to chill the tonic.

4. Garnish with a lemon slice or mint leaves for an extra refreshing touch.

5. Sip the ginseng tonic slowly and feel the mental clarity and sustained energy kick in.

4. Revitalizing Maca Mocha:

Ingredients:

- 1 teaspoon maca powder

- 1 cup brewed coffee, cooled

- 1/4 cup unsweetened almond milk (or milk of choice)

- 1 teaspoon cocoa powder

- 1 teaspoon honey or maple syrup (optional)

- Pinch of cinnamon

Instructions:

1. In a glass, combine the maca powder, brewed coffee, almond milk, cocoa powder, and honey or maple syrup (if using).

2. Stir the mixture until the ingredients are well incorporated.

3. Sprinkle a pinch of cinnamon on top for added flavor and aroma.

4. Serve the maca mocha chilled or over ice for a refreshing afternoon pick-me-up.

5. Enjoy the rich and creamy flavor of this revitalizing elixir as it boosts your energy and mood.

5. Refreshing Herbal Infusion:

Ingredients:

- 1 tablespoon dried herbs (such as peppermint, lemon balm, or chamomile)

- 1 cup boiling water

- 1 teaspoon honey or maple syrup (optional)

- Squeeze of fresh lemon juice

Instructions:

1. Place the dried herbs in a teapot or heatproof glass.

2. Pour the boiling water over the herbs and let steep for 5-10 minutes.

3. Strain the herbal infusion into a mug and discard the herbs.

4. Stir in the honey or maple syrup (if using) and add a squeeze of fresh lemon juice for extra flavor.

5. Sip the herbal infusion slowly and enjoy the soothing and refreshing benefits.

Tips for Enjoying Herbal Elixirs:

- Customize the elixirs according to your taste preferences by adjusting the sweetness or adding additional flavorings such as vanilla or cinnamon.

- Experiment with different adaptogenic herbs such as rhodiola, holy basil, or cordyceps to find the blend that works best for you.

- Enjoy your herbal elixirs as a mid-afternoon snack or as a refreshing beverage to accompany your afternoon activities.

- Incorporate herbal elixirs into your daily routine to support sustained energy, mental clarity, and overall well-being.

By incorporating these invigorating herbal elixirs into your afternoon routine, you can sustain your energy levels, support mental focus, and enhance your overall vitality. Cheers to revitalizing afternoons with nourishing herbal goodness!

CHAPTER EIGHT

Evening Relaxation: Unwind and Cleanse with Soothing Herbal Concoctions

As the day comes to a close, it's essential to take time to unwind, relax, and cleanse both the body and mind. Herbal concoctions offer a gentle and soothing way to promote relaxation, support digestion, and prepare the body for restful sleep. In this guide, we'll explore some calming herbal concoctions designed to help you unwind and cleanse in the evening.

1. Soothing Chamomile Lavender Tea:

Ingredients:

- 1 tablespoon dried chamomile flowers

- 1 teaspoon dried lavender buds

- 1 cup boiling water

- 1 teaspoon honey or maple syrup (optional)

- Squeeze of fresh lemon juice

Instructions:

1. Place the dried chamomile flowers and lavender buds in a teapot or heatproof glass.

2. Pour the boiling water over the herbs and let steep for 5-10 minutes.

3. Strain the tea into a mug and discard the herbs.

4. Stir in the honey or maple syrup (if using) and add a squeeze of fresh lemon juice for extra flavor.

5. Sip the chamomile lavender tea slowly and feel the calming effects wash over you as you unwind for the evening.

2. Relaxing Lemon Balm Mint Infusion:

Ingredients:

- 1 tablespoon dried lemon balm leaves

- 1 tablespoon fresh mint leaves

- 1 cup boiling water

- 1 teaspoon honey or maple syrup (optional)

- Squeeze of fresh lemon juice

Instructions:

1. Place the dried lemon balm leaves and fresh mint leaves in a teapot or heatproof glass.

2. Pour the boiling water over the herbs and let steep for 5-10 minutes.

3. Strain the infusion into a mug and discard the herbs.

4. Stir in the honey or maple syrup (if using) and add a squeeze of fresh lemon juice for a burst of flavor.

5. Sip the lemon balm mint infusion slowly and enjoy the soothing and refreshing benefits as you wind down for the evening.

3. Digestive Detox Turmeric Ginger Tonic:

Ingredients:

- 1-inch piece of fresh turmeric (peeled and grated)

- 1-inch piece of fresh ginger (peeled and grated)

- 1 tablespoon fresh lemon juice

- 1 teaspoon raw honey or maple syrup

- Pinch of ground cinnamon

- 1 cup warm water

Instructions:

1. In a mug, combine the grated turmeric and ginger with the fresh lemon juice, raw honey or maple syrup, and ground cinnamon.

2. Pour the warm water over the mixture and stir until the ingredients are well combined.

3. Allow the tonic to steep for a few minutes to infuse the flavors.

4. Sip the turmeric ginger tonic slowly and feel the gentle warmth and cleansing effects soothe your digestive system and prepare you for a restful night's sleep.

4. Herbal Sleepytime Elixir:

Ingredients:

- 1 tablespoon dried valerian root

- 1 tablespoon dried passionflower

- 1 tablespoon dried chamomile flowers

- 1 cup boiling water

- 1 teaspoon raw honey or maple syrup (optional)

Instructions:

1. Place the dried valerian root, passionflower, and chamomile flowers in a teapot or heatproof glass.

2. Pour the boiling water over the herbs and let steep for 10-15 minutes.

3. Strain the elixir into a mug and discard the herbs.

4. Stir in the raw honey or maple syrup (if using) for a touch of sweetness.

5. Sip the herbal sleepytime elixir slowly and feel the calming and sedative effects gently lull you into a state of relaxation and tranquility.

5. Cleansing Herbal Detox Broth:

Ingredients:

- 4 cups water
- 1-inch piece of fresh ginger (peeled and sliced)
- 1 garlic clove (crushed)
- 1 tablespoon dried burdock root
- 1 tablespoon dried dandelion root
- 1 tablespoon dried nettle leaf
- 1 tablespoon dried cleavers
- Salt and pepper to taste

Instructions:

1. In a large pot, bring the water to a boil.
2. Add the sliced ginger, crushed garlic clove, dried burdock root, dried dandelion root, dried nettle leaf, and dried cleavers to the pot.
3. Reduce the heat and simmer the broth for 20-30 minutes, allowing the herbs to infuse into the water.

4. Strain the broth into mugs and season with salt and pepper to taste.

5. Sip the herbal detox broth slowly and feel the cleansing and purifying effects support your body's natural detoxification processes as you prepare for a restful night's sleep.

Tips for Enjoying Evening Herbal Concoctions:

- Create a calming evening ritual by enjoying your herbal concoction in a quiet and peaceful environment, free from distractions.

- Take slow, deep breaths as you sip your herbal concoction to enhance relaxation and promote mindfulness.

- Customize your herbal concoctions by experimenting with different herbs, spices, and flavorings to suit your taste preferences and health goals.

- Incorporate herbal concoctions into your nightly routine to support relaxation, digestion, and restful sleep on a consistent basis.

By incorporating these soothing and cleansing herbal concoctions into your evening routine, you can promote relaxation, support digestion, and prepare your body and mind for a restful night's sleep. Cheers to peaceful evenings and rejuvenating nights with nourishing herbal goodness!

CHAPTER NINE

Weekly Meal Plans: Structuring Your Cleanse for Optimal Results

Embarking on a cleanse requires thoughtful planning to ensure you're nourishing your body with the right foods and supporting its natural detoxification processes. Structuring your cleanse with a well-designed weekly meal plan can help you stay on track, maximize results, and optimize your overall health and well-being. In this guide, we'll outline a sample weekly meal plan for a cleanse, including breakfast, lunch, dinner, and snacks, to help you achieve optimal results.

Day 1: Detox Kickoff

Breakfast:
Green smoothie with spinach, kale, banana, and coconut water

Snack:
Sliced cucumber and carrot sticks with hummus

Lunch:
Quinoa salad with mixed greens, cherry tomatoes, cucumber, avocado, and lemon-tahini dressing

Snack:

Fresh berries (such as strawberries, blueberries, raspberries)

Dinner:

Grilled salmon with steamed broccoli and quinoa *Evening Beverage:* Chamomile lavender tea

Day 2: Energizing Cleanse

Breakfast:

Acai berry smoothie bowl with granola, sliced banana, and chia seeds

Snack:

Green apple slices with almond butter

Lunch:

Zucchini noodles with marinara sauce and chickpea "meatballs"

Snack:

Celery sticks with almond butter and raisins (ants on a log)

Dinner:
Stir-fried tofu with mixed vegetables (bell peppers, snap peas, carrots) in a ginger-garlic sauce served over brown rice
Evening *Beverage:*
Turmeric golden milk latte

Day 3: Cleansing Vitality

Breakfast:
Detoxifying green juice with cucumber, celery, kale, lemon, ginger, and parsley

Snack:
Raw almonds and pumpkin seeds

Lunch:
Roasted sweet potato and black bean salad with avocado, cherry tomatoes, and cilantro-lime dressing

Snack:
Sliced pineapple and mango

Dinner:
Baked cod with roasted Brussels sprouts and quinoa pilaf

Evening   *Beverage:*

Peppermint herbal infusion

Day 4: Rejuvenating Balance

Breakfast:

Chia seed pudding made with almond milk, topped with mixed berries and shredded coconut

Snack:

Carrot and cucumber sticks with tzatziki sauce

Lunch:

Lentil soup with kale, carrots, celery, and turmeric

Snack:

Sliced pear with almond butter

Dinner:

Grilled chicken breast with roasted asparagus and cauliflower mash

Evening   *Beverage:*

Lemon ginger detox water

Day 5: Nourishing Renewal

Breakfast:
Oatmeal topped with sliced banana, walnuts, and cinnamon

Snack:
Raw cashews and dried apricots

Lunch:
Mediterranean quinoa salad with cherry tomatoes, cucumber, Kalamata olives, feta cheese, and lemon-herb vinaigrette

Snack:
Sliced bell peppers with guacamole

Dinner:
Vegetable stir-fry with tofu or tempeh in a teriyaki sauce served over brown rice
Evening *Beverage:*
Chamomile lavender tea

Day 6: Balancing Harmony

Breakfast:

Smoothie bowl with mixed berries, banana, spinach, almond milk, and hemp seeds

Snack:

Trail mix with mixed nuts, seeds, and dried fruit

Lunch:

Quinoa tabbouleh salad with cucumber, tomato, parsley, mint, and lemon-tahini dressing

Snack:

Sliced cucumber and cherry tomatoes with balsamic glaze

Dinner:

Grilled shrimp skewers with roasted vegetables (zucchini, bell peppers, onions) and quinoa

Evening Beverage:

Turmeric golden milk latte

Day 7: Restorative Renewal

Breakfast:
Avocado toast on whole grain bread with sliced tomato and arugula

Snack:
Apple slices with almond butter

Lunch:
Kale and white bean soup with garlic, onion, carrots, celery, and vegetable broth

Snack:
Mixed berry smoothie with almond milk and protein powder

Dinner:
Baked salmon with roasted sweet potatoes and steamed broccoli

Evening   Beverage:
Peppermint herbal infusion

Tips for Success:

1. **Stay Hydrated:** Drink plenty of water throughout the day to support hydration and detoxification.

2. **Listen to Your Body:** Pay attention to how different foods make you feel and adjust your meal plan accordingly.

3. **Incorporate Variety:** Include a wide variety of fruits, vegetables, whole grains, legumes, nuts, seeds, and lean proteins in your meals to ensure you're getting a diverse range of nutrients.

4. **Practice Mindful Eating:** Take the time to savor and enjoy your meals, paying attention to flavors, textures, and sensations.

5. **Get Adequate Rest:** Prioritize quality sleep to support your body's natural cleansing and rejuvenation processes.

6. **Move Your Body:** Incorporate gentle exercise such as walking, yoga, or stretching to support circulation, digestion, and overall well-being.

By structuring your cleanse with a well-designed weekly meal plan, you can support your body's natural detoxification processes, nourish your cells with essential nutrients, and achieve optimal results for your health and well-being. Cheers to a week of cleansing and revitalization!

CHAPTER TEN

Beyond the Cleanse: Integrating Herbal Juicing into a Healthy Lifestyle

Herbal juicing offers a myriad of health benefits beyond just cleansing, making it a valuable addition to a healthy lifestyle. By incorporating herbal juices into your daily routine, you can nourish your body with essential nutrients, support detoxification, boost energy levels, and enhance overall well-being. In this guide, we'll explore how to integrate herbal juicing into a sustainable and balanced healthy lifestyle for long-term health and vitality.

1. Make Herbal Juicing a Daily Habit:

Commit to making herbal juicing a daily habit by incorporating it into your morning routine. Start your day with a revitalizing herbal juice to kickstart your metabolism, hydrate your body, and flood your cells with essential vitamins, minerals, and antioxidants. Experiment with different herbal juice recipes to keep things interesting and explore the wide variety of flavors and health benefits that herbal juicing has to offer.

2. Choose Quality Ingredients:

Selecting high-quality, organic ingredients is essential for maximizing the nutritional value and health benefits of your herbal juices. Choose fresh, locally sourced fruits, vegetables, and herbs whenever possible to ensure you're getting the highest quality ingredients. Opt for organic produce to minimize exposure to pesticides and chemicals, and wash fruits and vegetables thoroughly before juicing to remove any dirt or residue.

3. Focus on Variety and Balance:

Incorporate a diverse range of fruits, vegetables, and herbs into your herbal juices to ensure you're getting a wide spectrum of nutrients and health-promoting compounds. Experiment with different combinations of ingredients to create delicious and nutrient-rich juice blends that appeal to your taste buds and support your health goals. Aim to include a balance of leafy greens, colorful fruits and vegetables, herbs, and superfoods in your herbal juices for optimal nutrition and flavor.

4. Listen to Your Body:

Pay attention to how your body responds to different herbal juices and adjust your recipes accordingly to meet your individual needs and preferences. Notice how certain ingredients make you feel and incorporate those that leave you feeling energized, refreshed, and nourished. Be mindful of any sensitivities or intolerances you may have to specific ingredients and choose alternatives that work best for you.

5. Incorporate Herbal Juices into Meals:

Integrate herbal juices into your meals as a refreshing beverage or accompaniment to your favorite dishes. Enjoy a glass of herbal juice alongside breakfast, lunch, or dinner to hydrate your body and enhance the flavor and nutritional content of your meals. Consider pairing herbal juices with nutrient-dense foods such as salads, smoothie bowls, grain bowls, or lean proteins for a complete and balanced meal.

6. Prioritize Whole Foods:

While herbal juices can be a convenient way to boost your intake of vitamins, minerals, and antioxidants, it's important to prioritize whole foods as the foundation of a healthy diet. Use herbal juices to complement a diet rich in whole, unprocessed foods such as fruits, vegetables, whole grains, legumes, nuts, seeds, and lean proteins. Aim to consume a variety of nutrient-dense foods from all food groups to ensure you're meeting your nutritional needs and supporting overall health and well-being.

7. Practice Moderation:

While herbal juices can be a beneficial addition to a healthy lifestyle, it's important to practice moderation and avoid excessive consumption. While fresh juices can provide essential nutrients and hydration, they can also be high in natural sugars and calories, especially when made with sweet fruits. Enjoy herbal juices as part of a balanced diet and lifestyle, but be mindful of portion sizes and avoid relying on them as the sole source of nutrition.

8. Stay Hydrated:

In addition to herbal juices, prioritize hydration by drinking plenty of water throughout the day. Water is essential for supporting digestion, circulation, detoxification, and overall cellular function. Aim to drink at least 8-10 glasses of water per day, and hydrate your body with herbal juices, herbal teas, coconut water, and other hydrating beverages to maintain optimal hydration levels.

By integrating herbal juicing into a healthy lifestyle, you can nourish your body with essential nutrients, support detoxification, boost energy levels, and enhance overall well-being. Embrace herbal juicing as a delicious and convenient way to promote health and vitality for long-term wellness. Cheers to a vibrant and balanced lifestyle with herbal goodness!

CHAPTER 11

SOME HERBAL JUICE RECIPES FOR MUCUS CLEANSE

1. **Peppermint Lemonade:**

   - **Definition:** Peppermint is known for its soothing properties, while lemon helps in detoxifying the body.

   - **Ingredients:** Peppermint leaves, lemon juice, honey (optional), water.

   - **Preparation:** Blend peppermint leaves with lemon juice and water. Add honey for sweetness.

   - **How to Use:** Drink it throughout the day.

   - **Dosage:** 1-2 glasses daily.

   - **Side Effects:** Peppermint may cause heartburn in some individuals.

2. **Ginger Turmeric Tea:**

   - **Definition:** Ginger and turmeric have anti-inflammatory properties that can help in reducing mucus.

   - **Ingredients:** Fresh ginger root, turmeric powder, lemon, honey (optional), water.

- **Preparation:** Boil sliced ginger and turmeric powder in water. Add lemon and honey.

- **How to Use:** Drink it warm.

- **Dosage:** 1-2 cups daily.

- **Side Effects:** May cause acidity in some cases.

3. Eucalyptus Tea:

- **Definition:** Eucalyptus is known for its decongestant properties.

- **Ingredients:** Eucalyptus leaves, honey (optional), water.

- **Preparation:** Steep eucalyptus leaves in hot water. Add honey if desired.

- **How to Use:** Drink it warm.

- **Dosage:** 1-2 cups daily.

- **Side Effects:** Excessive consumption may lead to nausea.

4. Nettle Leaf Infusion:

- **Definition:** Nettle leaf is a natural antihistamine and helps in reducing mucus production.

- **Ingredients:** Dried nettle leaves, water.

- **Preparation:** Steep dried nettle leaves in hot water for 10-15 minutes.

- **How to Use:** Drink it warm.

- **Dosage:** 1-2 cups daily.

- **Side Effects:** May cause allergic reactions in some individuals.

5. Garlic Lemon Elixir:

- **Definition:** Garlic has antimicrobial properties while lemon helps in detoxification.

- **Ingredients:** Garlic cloves, lemon juice, honey (optional), water.

- **Preparation:** Blend garlic cloves with lemon juice and water. Add honey for taste.

- **How to Use:** Drink it in the morning on an empty stomach.

- **Dosage:** 1 glass daily.

- **Side Effects:** May cause bad breath and stomach upset in some cases.

6. Fenugreek Seed Decoction:

- **Definition:** Fenugreek helps in loosening and expelling mucus from the respiratory tract.

- **Ingredients:** Fenugreek seeds, water.

- **Preparation:** Boil fenugreek seeds in water until it reduces to half.

- **How to Use:** Drink it warm.

- **Dosage:** 1-2 cups daily.

- **Side Effects:** May cause diarrhea or allergic reactions.

7. Licorice Root Tea:

- **Definition:** Licorice root has expectorant properties, helping to expel mucus.

- **Ingredients:** Licorice root, water.

- **Preparation:** Steep licorice root in hot water for 10-15 minutes.

- **How to Use:** Drink it warm.

- **Dosage:** 1-2 cups daily.

- **Side Effects:** Prolonged use may lead to high blood pressure.

8. Pineapple Celery Juice:

- **Definition:** Pineapple contains bromelain, which aids in breaking down mucus, and celery is hydrating.

- **Ingredients:** Pineapple, celery stalks.

- **Preparation:** Juice pineapple and celery together.

- **How to Use:** Drink it fresh.

- **Dosage:** 1 glass daily.

- **Side Effects:** Excessive consumption may cause digestive issues.

9. Horseradish Honey Tonic:

- **Definition:** Horseradish helps in clearing congestion, and honey soothes the throat.

- **Ingredients:** Grated horseradish, honey, water.

- **Preparation:** Mix grated horseradish with honey and water.

- **How to Use:** Take 1 tablespoon daily.

- **Dosage:** 1 tablespoon daily.

- **Side Effects:** May cause irritation in the mouth or digestive upset.

10. Dandelion Root Detox Juice:

- **Definition:** Dandelion root aids in liver detoxification, which can help reduce overall mucus production.

- **Ingredients:** Dandelion root, cucumber, lemon, water.

- **Preparation:** Juice dandelion root, cucumber, and lemon together.

- **How to Use:** Drink it fresh.

- **Dosage:** 1 glass daily.

- **Side Effects:** May cause allergic reactions in some individuals.

11.   **Chamomile Tea with Honey:**

- **Definition:** Chamomile has anti-inflammatory properties, and honey soothes the throat.

- **Ingredients:** Chamomile flowers, honey, water.

- **Preparation:** Steep chamomile flowers in hot water. Add honey for taste.

- **How to Use:** Drink it warm.

- **Dosage:** 1-2 cups daily.

- **Side Effects:** Rarely, may cause allergic reactions, especially in those allergic to ragweed.

12.   **Thyme Infusion:**

- **Definition:** Thyme is a natural expectorant and antimicrobial herb.

- **Ingredients:** Fresh thyme leaves, water.

- **Preparation:** Steep fresh thyme leaves in hot water for 10-15 minutes.

- **How to Use:** Drink it warm.

- **Dosage:** 1-2 cups daily.

- **Side Effects:** May cause allergic reactions or upset stomach in some individuals.

13.   **Cayenne Pepper Lemonade:**

- **Definition:** Cayenne pepper helps in clearing congestion and promoting circulation.

- **Ingredients:** Cayenne pepper, lemon juice, honey (optional), water.

- **Preparation:** Mix cayenne pepper, lemon juice, and honey in water.

- **How to Use:** Drink it throughout the day.

- **Dosage:** 1-2 glasses daily.

- **Side Effects:** May cause stomach upset or irritation in some individuals.

14.   **Burdock Root Cleanse Juice:**

- **Definition:** Burdock root helps in detoxification and improving lymphatic drainage.

- **Ingredients:** Burdock root, apple, lemon, water.

- **Preparation:** Juice burdock root, apple, and lemon together.

- **How to Use:** Drink it fresh.

- **Dosage:** 1 glass daily.

- **Side Effects:** Rarely, may cause allergic reactions.

15.   **Rosemary Mint Tea:**

- **Definition:** Rosemary and mint have decongestant properties and can help in clearing mucus.

- **Ingredients:** Fresh rosemary, fresh mint leaves, water.

- **Preparation:** Steep fresh rosemary and mint leaves in hot water for 10-15 minutes.

- **How to Use:** Drink it warm.

- **Dosage:** 1-2 cups daily.

- **Side Effects:** Rarely, may cause allergic reactions or upset stomach.

SOME HERBAL REMEDIES YOU NEED TO KNOW

Cascara Sagrada:

Definition: Cascara Sagrada, scientifically known as Rhamnus purshiana, is a species of buckthorn native to western North America. It has been used traditionally as a laxative and to promote bowel regularity.

Ingredients: The primary active ingredients in cascara sagrada are anthraquinone glycosides, particularly cascarosides A and B. These compounds stimulate peristalsis in the colon, leading to increased bowel movements.

How to Prepare: Cascara sagrada is typically prepared as an herbal tea, tincture, or capsule. To make tea, dried cascara sagrada bark is steeped in hot water for several minutes before being strained and consumed. Tinctures are prepared by steeping the bark in alcohol to extract its active compounds.

Dosage: The appropriate dosage of cascara sagrada can vary depending on the specific preparation and intended use. It's important to follow the recommended dosage on the product label or consult with a healthcare professional for personalized guidance.

How to Use: Cascara sagrada tea or tincture is typically taken orally. It's important to start with a low dose and gradually increase if needed to avoid potential side effects such as cramping or diarrhea.

Side Effects: Cascara sagrada is considered safe for short-term use when used as directed. However, long-term or excessive use may lead to dependence, electrolyte imbalance, or dehydration. It may also interact with certain medications or have adverse effects in individuals with certain health conditions. It's important to use cascara sagrada under the guidance of a healthcare professional and to discontinue use if any adverse effects occur.

Cell Food:

Definition: Cell Food is a dietary supplement marketed as a highly oxygenating and alkalizing formula. It's claimed to support overall health and vitality by providing essential nutrients and oxygen to the cells.

Ingredients: The exact ingredients of Cell Food can vary depending on the brand, but it typically contains a proprietary blend of minerals, enzymes, electrolytes, and trace elements. Some common ingredients may include purified water, dissolved oxygen, seawater extract, and plant-based enzymes.

How to Prepare: Cell Food is usually available in liquid form and is typically taken orally. It can be consumed directly or diluted in water or juice before consumption.

Dosage: The dosage of Cell Food can vary depending on the specific product and individual needs. It's important to follow the recommended dosage on the product label or consult with a healthcare professional for personalized guidance.

How to Use: Cell Food is typically taken orally, either directly or mixed into water or juice. It's important to shake the bottle well before use and to store it according to the manufacturer's instructions.

Side Effects: Cell Food is generally considered safe for most people when used as directed. However, some individuals may experience mild digestive upset or allergic reactions to certain ingredients. It's essential to consult with a healthcare provider before starting any new supplement regimen, especially if you have underlying health conditions or are taking medications.

Chaparral:

Definition: Chaparral, scientifically known as Larrea tridentata, is a shrub native to the southwestern United States and northern Mexico. It has been used for centuries by Native American tribes for its medicinal properties and is commonly used in herbal medicine today.

Ingredients: Chaparral contains several bioactive compounds, including nordihydroguaiaretic acid (NDGA), flavonoids, lignans, and volatile oils. NDGA is believed to be the primary active compound responsible for many of chaparral's therapeutic effects.

How to Prepare: Chaparral can be prepared and consumed in various forms, including teas, tinctures, capsules, and topical preparations. To make tea, dried chaparral leaves are steeped in hot water for several minutes before being strained and consumed. Tinctures are prepared by steeping the herb in alcohol or vinegar to extract its active compounds.

Dosage: The appropriate dosage of chaparral can vary depending on the specific form and intended use. It's important to follow the recommended dosage on the product label or consult with a healthcare professional for personalized guidance.

How to Use: Chaparral tea or tincture is typically taken orally. It can also be applied topically to the skin for certain conditions. It's important to use chaparral products as directed and to discontinue use if any adverse effects occur.

Side Effects: Chaparral is generally considered safe for most people when used in moderate amounts. However, excessive intake or prolonged use may lead to liver toxicity or other adverse effects. It may also interact with certain medications or have adverse effects in individuals with certain health conditions. It's important to use chaparral under the guidance of a healthcare professional and to discontinue use if any adverse effects occur.

Cocolmeca:

Definition: Cocolmeca, also known as Smilax ornata or sarsaparilla, is a flowering vine native to Mexico and Central America. It has been used traditionally in Mexican and Central American folk medicine for its purported medicinal properties.

Ingredients: Cocolmeca contains various bioactive compounds, including saponins, flavonoids, and plant sterols. These compounds are believed to contribute to the herb's medicinal properties, including its potential as a diuretic, blood purifier, and anti-inflammatory agent.

How to Prepare: Cocolmeca is commonly prepared and consumed as an herbal tea or decoction. To make tea, dried cocolmeca roots or leaves are steeped in hot water for several minutes before being strained and consumed. Decoctions involve boiling the roots or leaves in water to extract their active compounds.

Dosage: The appropriate dosage of cocolmeca can vary depending on factors such as age, health status, and the specific preparation being used. It's important to follow the recommended dosage on the product label or consult with a qualified herbalist or healthcare professional for personalized guidance.

How to Use: Cocolmeca tea or decoction is typically taken orally. It can also be used topically for certain skin conditions. It's important to use cocolmeca products as directed and to discontinue use if any adverse effects occur.

Side Effects: Cocolmeca is generally considered safe for most people when used in moderate amounts. However, excessive intake may lead to digestive upset or other adverse effects. It may also interact with certain medications or have adverse effects in individuals with certain health conditions. It's important to use cocolmeca under the guidance of a healthcare professional and to discontinue use if any adverse effects occur.

Contribo:

Definition: Contribo, also known as Aristolochiatrilobata, is a vine native to the Caribbean and Central America. It has been used traditionally in folk medicine for various purposes, including as a remedy for digestive issues, inflammation, and pain relief.

Ingredients: Contribo contains several bioactive compounds, including aristolochic acids, flavonoids, and alkaloids. These compounds are believed to contribute to the herb's medicinal properties, including its potential as an anti-inflammatory and analgesic agent.

How to Prepare: Contribo is typically prepared and consumed as an herbal tea or decoction. To make tea, dried contribo leaves or stems are steeped in hot water for several minutes before being strained and consumed. Decoctions involve boiling the leaves or stems in water to extract their active compounds.

Dosage: The appropriate dosage of contribo can vary depending on factors such as age, health status, and the specific preparation being used. It's important to follow the recommended dosage on the product label or consult with a qualified herbalist or healthcare professional for personalized guidance.

How to Use: Contribo tea or decoction is typically taken orally. It's important to use contribo products as directed and to discontinue use if any adverse effects occur.

Side Effects: Contribo contains aristolochic acids, which have been associated with serious adverse effects, including kidney damage and cancer. Due to these safety concerns, the use of contribo is highly discouraged, and it's important to avoid products containing aristolochic acids. Individuals should seek alternative remedies for their health needs.

Dandelion Root:

Definition: Dandelion, scientifically known as Taraxacum officinale, is a common flowering plant found worldwide. While often considered a pesky weed, dandelion has a long history of use in traditional medicine for its various health benefits.

Ingredients: Dandelion root contains several bioactive compounds, including sesquiterpene lactones, triterpenes, flavonoids, and polysaccharides. These compounds are believed to contribute to the herb's medicinal properties, including its potential as a diuretic, digestive aid, and liver tonic.

How to Prepare: Dandelion root can be prepared and consumed in various forms, including teas, tinctures, capsules, and extracts. To make tea, dried dandelion root is steeped in hot water for several minutes before being strained and consumed. Tinctures are prepared by steeping the root in alcohol or vinegar to extract its active compounds.

Dosage: The appropriate dosage of dandelion root can vary depending on factors such as age, health status, and the specific preparation being used. It's important to follow the recommended dosage on the product label or consult with a qualified herbalist or healthcare professional for personalized guidance.

How to Use: Dandelion root tea, tincture, or capsules are typically taken orally. It's important to use dandelion root products as directed and to discontinue use if any adverse effects occur.

Side Effects: Dandelion root is generally considered safe for most people when used in moderate amounts. However, some individuals may experience allergic reactions or digestive upset. It may also interact with certain medications or have adverse effects in individuals with certain health conditions. It's important to use dandelion root under the guidance of a healthcare professional and to discontinue use if any adverse effects occur.

Green Food Plus:

Definition: Green Food Plus is a dietary supplement formulated to provide a concentrated source of nutrients derived from various green plants. It's designed to support overall health and well-being by delivering essential vitamins, minerals, antioxidants, and phytonutrients.

Ingredients: Green Food Plus typically contains a blend of powdered green vegetables, grasses, algae, and other plant-based ingredients. Common ingredients may include wheatgrass, barley grass, spirulina, chlorella, alfalfa, kale, spinach, and broccoli, among others.

How to Prepare: Green Food Plus is usually available in powder form and can be mixed with water, juice, or smoothies. It's important to follow the recommended dosage on the product label and to consume it as part of a balanced diet.

Dosage: The appropriate dosage of Green Food Plus can vary depending on the specific product and individual needs. It's important to follow the recommended dosage on the product label or consult with a healthcare professional for personalized guidance.

How to Use: Green Food Plus powder is typically mixed with water, juice, or smoothies and consumed orally. It's often taken once or twice daily, preferably with meals, to maximize nutrient absorption.

Side Effects: Green Food Plus is generally considered safe for most people when used as directed. However, some individuals may experience digestive upset or allergic reactions to certain ingredients. It's important to consult with a healthcare provider before starting any new supplement regimen, especially if you have underlying health conditions or are taking medications.

Guaco:

Definition: Guaco, also known as Mikania cordata or Mikania glomerata, is a medicinal plant native to Central and South America. It has a long history of use in traditional medicine for its potential therapeutic properties.

Ingredients: Guaco contains several bioactive compounds, including coumarins, flavonoids, tannins, and saponins. These compounds are believed to contribute to the herb's medicinal properties, including its potential as an expectorant, anti-inflammatory, and antispasmodic agent.

How to Prepare: Guaco is typically prepared and consumed as an herbal tea or infusion. To make tea, dried guaco leaves are steeped in hot water for several minutes before being strained and consumed.

Dosage: The appropriate dosage of guaco can vary depending on factors such as age, health status, and the specific preparation being used. It's important to follow the recommended dosage on the product label or consult with a qualified herbalist or healthcare professional for personalized guidance.

How to Use: Guaco tea is typically taken orally. It can be consumed on its own or mixed with honey or other herbal teas for added flavor.

Side Effects: Guaco is generally considered safe for most people when used in moderate amounts. However, some individuals may experience allergic reactions or digestive upset. It may also interact with certain medications or have adverse effects in individuals with certain health conditions. It's important to use guaco under the guidance of a healthcare professional and to discontinue use if any adverse effects occur.

Herban Iron:

Definition: Herban Iron is a dietary supplement designed to provide an easily absorbable form of iron to support healthy iron levels in the body. It's particularly beneficial for individuals with iron deficiency or anemia.

Ingredients: Herban Iron typically contains iron in the form of ferrous bisglycinate, which is a highly bioavailable and gentle form of iron that is less likely to cause digestive upset or constipation compared to other forms of iron. It may also contain other ingredients such as vitamin C to enhance iron absorption.

How to Prepare: Herban Iron is usually available in capsule or liquid form. Capsules are taken orally with water, while liquid forms may be mixed with water or juice before consumption. It's important to follow the recommended dosage on the product label.

Dosage: The appropriate dosage of Herban Iron depends on factors such as age, gender, and the severity of iron deficiency. It's important to consult with a healthcare professional to determine the correct dosage for individual needs.

How to Use: Herban Iron capsules are typically taken orally with water, while liquid forms may be mixed with water or juice before consumption. It's important to take Herban Iron as directed and to avoid taking it with dairy products, antacids, or other substances that may interfere with iron absorption.

Side Effects: While Herban Iron is generally considered safe for most people when used as directed, some individuals may experience mild side effects such as gastrointestinal discomfort or constipation. It's important to consult with a healthcare professional before starting any new supplement regimen, especially if you have underlying health conditions or are taking medications.

Hydrangea:

Definition: Hydrangea, scientifically known as Hydrangea arborescens, is a flowering shrub native to North America. It has been used traditionally in herbal medicine for its potential diuretic and anti-inflammatory properties.

Ingredients: Hydrangea contains several bioactive compounds, including saponins, flavonoids, and glycosides. These compounds are believed to contribute to the herb's medicinal properties, including its potential as a diuretic, kidney tonic, and anti-inflammatory agent.

How to Prepare: Hydrangea root is typically prepared and consumed as an herbal tea or tincture. To make tea, dried hydrangea root is steeped in hot water for several minutes before being strained and consumed. Tinctures are prepared by steeping the root in alcohol or vinegar to extract its active compounds.

Dosage: The appropriate dosage of hydrangea can vary depending on factors such as age, health status, and the specific preparation being used. It's important to follow the recommended dosage on the product label or consult with a qualified herbalist or healthcare professional for personalized guidance.

How to Use: Hydrangea tea or tincture is typically taken orally. It's important to use hydrangea products as directed and to discontinue use if any adverse effects occur.

Side Effects: Hydrangea is generally considered safe for most people when used in moderate amounts. However, some individuals may experience digestive upset or allergic reactions. It may also interact with certain medications or have adverse effects in individuals with certain health conditions. It's important to use hydrangea under the guidance of a healthcare professional and to discontinue use if any adverse effects occur.

Irish Moss:

Definition: Irish Moss, scientifically known as Chondrus crispus, is a species of red algae or seaweed native to the Atlantic coastlines of Europe and North America. It has been used for centuries in traditional Irish and Scottish cuisine, as well as in herbal medicine.

Ingredients: Irish Moss is rich in various nutrients, including iodine, sulfur compounds, vitamins (such as vitamin A, vitamin K, and vitamin B12), minerals (including calcium, magnesium, potassium, and sodium), and polysaccharides (such as carrageenan). These nutrients are believed to contribute to the herb's potential health benefits.

How to Prepare: Irish Moss is typically prepared by soaking it in water to rehydrate and soften it before use. It can be added to soups, stews, smoothies, desserts, and other dishes as a thickening agent or nutritional supplement.

Dosage: The appropriate dosage of Irish Moss can vary depending on factors such as age, health status, and the specific preparation being used. It's important to follow recipes or guidelines for culinary use and to consult with a healthcare professional for guidance on using Irish Moss as a dietary supplement.

How to Use: Irish Moss can be used in culinary applications to add thickness and nutritional value to dishes. It can also be consumed as a dietary supplement in the form of capsules, powders, or extracts.

Side Effects: Irish Moss is generally considered safe for most people when consumed in moderate amounts as part of a balanced diet. However, some individuals may be allergic to seaweed or carrageenan, a compound found in Irish Moss that is used as a food additive. It's important to discontinue use if any adverse effects occur and to consult with a healthcare professional if you have any concerns.

Red Clover:

Definition: Red clover, scientifically known as Trifolium pratense, is a flowering plant belonging to the legume family. It's native to Europe, Western Asia, and Northwest Africa but has been naturalized in many other regions. Red clover has been used in traditional medicine for various purposes, including its potential to support women's health and menopausal symptoms.

Ingredients: Red clover contains several bioactive compounds, including isoflavones (such as genistein and daidzein), flavonoids, and phytoestrogens. These compounds are believed to contribute to the herb's medicinal properties, including its potential as a hormone-balancing agent and its ability to support cardiovascular health.

How to Prepare: Red clover is typically prepared and consumed as an herbal tea or tincture. To make tea, dried red clover flowers are steeped in hot water for several minutes before being strained and consumed. Tinctures are prepared by steeping the flowers in alcohol or vinegar to extract their active compounds.

Dosage: The appropriate dosage of red clover can vary depending on factors such as age, health status, and the specific preparation being used. It's important to follow the recommended dosage on the product label or consult with a qualified herbalist or healthcare professional for personalized guidance.

How to Use: Red clover tea or tincture is typically taken orally. It's important to use red clover products as directed and to discontinue use if any adverse effects occur.

Side Effects: Red clover is generally considered safe for most people when used in moderate amounts. However, some individuals may experience allergic reactions or digestive upset. It may also interact with certain medications or have adverse effects in individuals with certain health conditions. It's important to use red clover under the guidance of a healthcare professional and to discontinue use if any adverse effects occur.

Sarsaparilla:

Definition: Sarsaparilla refers to several species of plants belonging to the Smilax genus, including Smilax regelii and Smilax officinalis. It has been used historically in traditional medicine for its potential health benefits, particularly for its purported detoxifying and anti-inflammatory properties.

Ingredients: Sarsaparilla contains various bioactive compounds, including saponins (such as sarsaponin and smilagenin), flavonoids, phenolic acids, and sterols. These compounds are believed to contribute to the herb's medicinal properties, including its potential as a diuretic, blood purifier, and anti-inflammatory agent.

How to Prepare: Sarsaparilla root is typically prepared and consumed as an herbal tea, decoction, or tincture. To make tea, dried sarsaparilla root is steeped in hot water for several minutes before being strained and consumed. Decoctions involve boiling the root in water to extract its active compounds, while tinctures are prepared by steeping the root in alcohol or vinegar.

Dosage: The appropriate dosage of sarsaparilla can vary depending on factors such as age, health status, and the specific preparation being used. It's important to follow the recommended dosage on the product label or consult with a qualified herbalist or healthcare professional for personalized guidance.

How to Use: Sarsaparilla tea or tincture is typically taken orally. It's important to use sarsaparilla products as directed and to discontinue use if any adverse effects occur.

Side Effects: Sarsaparilla is generally considered safe for most people when used in moderate amounts. However, some individuals may experience allergic reactions or digestive upset. It may also interact with certain medications or have adverse effects in individuals with certain health conditions. It's important to use sarsaparilla under the guidance of a healthcare professional and to discontinue use if any adverse effects occur.

Tila:

Definition: Tila, also known as linden flower or lime blossom, refers to the flowers of the Tilia genus, primarily Tilia europaea and Tilia cordata. These trees are native to Europe, but they are also cultivated in other regions for their fragrant and medicinal flowers.

Ingredients: Tila flowers contain various bioactive compounds, including flavonoids, phenolic acids, and volatile oils. These compounds are believed to contribute to the herb's medicinal properties, including its potential as a mild sedative, anxiolytic, and anti-inflammatory agent.

How to Prepare: Tila flowers are typically prepared and consumed as an herbal tea or infusion. To make tea, dried tila flowers are steeped in hot water for several minutes before being strained and consumed.

Dosage: The appropriate dosage of tila can vary depending on factors such as age, health status, and the specific preparation being used. It's important to follow the recommended dosage on the product label or consult with a qualified herbalist or healthcare professional for personalized guidance.

How to Use: Tila tea is typically taken orally. It's often consumed in the evening as a calming bedtime beverage or during times of stress or anxiety. It's important to use tila products as directed and to discontinue use if any adverse effects occur.

Side Effects: Tila is generally considered safe for most people when used in moderate amounts. However, some individuals may experience allergic reactions or digestive upset. It may also interact with certain medications or have adverse effects in individuals with certain health conditions. It's important to use tila under the guidance of a healthcare professional and to discontinue use if any adverse effects occur.

Valerian:

Definition: Valerian, scientifically known as Valeriana officinalis, is a perennial flowering plant native to Europe and Asia. It has been used for centuries in traditional medicine for its potential calming and sedative effects.

Ingredients: Valerian root contains several bioactive compounds, including valerenic acid, valepotriates, and volatile oils. These compounds are believed to contribute to the herb's medicinal properties, including its potential as a sedative, anxiolytic, and sleep aid.

How to Prepare: Valerian root is typically prepared and consumed as an herbal tea, tincture, or capsule. To make tea, dried valerian root is steeped in hot water for several minutes before being strained and consumed. Tinctures are prepared by steeping the root in alcohol or vinegar to extract its active compounds.

Dosage: The appropriate dosage of valerian can vary depending on factors such as age, health status, and the specific preparation being used. It's important to follow the recommended dosage on the product label or consult with a qualified herbalist or healthcare professional for personalized guidance.

How to Use: Valerian tea, tincture, or capsules are typically taken orally. It's often consumed in the evening as a sleep aid or during times of stress or anxiety. It's important to use valerian products as directed and to discontinue use if any adverse effects occur.

Side Effects: Valerian is generally considered safe for most people when used in moderate amounts. However, some individuals may experience mild side effects such as drowsiness, headache, or gastrointestinal upset. It may also interact with certain medications or have adverse effects in individuals with certain health conditions. It's important to use valerian under the guidance of a healthcare professional and to discontinue use if any adverse effects occur.

Red Raspberry:

Definition: Red raspberry, scientifically known as Rubus idaeus, is a species of raspberry native to Europe and northern Asia. It's widely cultivated for its delicious berries and has been used in traditional medicine for various purposes, including its potential to support women's health during pregnancy and childbirth.

Ingredients: Red raspberry contains several bioactive compounds, including flavonoids, ellagic acid, anthocyanins, and vitamin C. These compounds are believed to contribute to the herb's medicinal properties, including its potential as an antioxidant, anti-inflammatory, and uterine tonic.

How to Prepare: Red raspberry leaf is typically prepared and consumed as an herbal tea or infusion. To make tea, dried red raspberry leaves are steeped in hot water for several minutes before being strained and consumed.

Dosage: The appropriate dosage of red raspberry leaf can vary depending on factors such as age, health status, and the specific preparation being used. It's important to follow the recommended dosage on the product label or consult with a qualified herbalist or healthcare professional for personalized guidance.

How to Use: Red raspberry leaf tea is typically taken orally. It's often recommended for pregnant individuals in the later stages of pregnancy to support uterine health and prepare for childbirth. It's important to use red raspberry leaf products as directed and to discontinue use if any adverse effects occur.

Side Effects: Red raspberry leaf is generally considered safe for most people when used in moderate amounts. However, some individuals may experience allergic reactions or digestive upset. Pregnant individuals should consult with a healthcare professional before using red raspberry leaf, especially if they have any underlying health conditions or are taking medications. It's important to use red raspberry leaf under the guidance of a healthcare professional and to discontinue use if any adverse effects occur.

Rhubarb:

Definition: Rhubarb, scientifically known as Rheum rhabarbarum, is a perennial plant cultivated for its edible stalks. While primarily used in culinary applications, rhubarb has also been utilized in traditional medicine for its potential health benefits, particularly for digestive health.

Ingredients: Rhubarb stalks contain various bioactive compounds, including anthraquinones (such as emodin and rhein), fiber, vitamins (such as vitamin K), and minerals (including calcium and potassium). These compounds are believed to contribute to the herb's medicinal properties, including its potential as a laxative and digestive aid.

How to Prepare: Rhubarb stalks are typically cooked before consumption, as the raw stalks are very tart and can be unpleasant to eat. They are often used in pies, crisps, jams, sauces, and other desserts, as well as in savory dishes. Rhubarb can also be used to make compotes, jams, and preserves.

Dosage: There is no specific dosage for rhubarb in culinary applications, as it is used as a food rather than a medicinal herb. However, when used for its potential laxative effects, it's important to consume rhubarb in moderation to avoid gastrointestinal upset.

How to Use: Rhubarb stalks can be chopped and cooked in various dishes, including pies, sauces, and jams. It's important to remove and discard the leaves, as they contain toxic compounds. When using rhubarb for its potential laxative effects, it's typically consumed as part of a cooked dish or in the form of a rhubarb-based herbal remedy.

Side Effects: Rhubarb stalks are generally safe for most people when consumed in moderate amounts as part of a balanced diet. However, excessive intake may lead to digestive upset or adverse effects due to the presence of oxalic acid, which can bind to calcium and form kidney stones in susceptible individuals. It's important to use rhubarb in moderation and to consult with a healthcare professional if you have any concerns or underlying health conditions.

Irish Sea Moss:

Definition: Irish Sea Moss is a term often used interchangeably with Irish Moss, referring to the same species of red algae, Chondrus crispus. It's harvested from the rocky shores of the Atlantic coastlines of Europe and North America.

Ingredients: Irish Sea Moss shares the same nutritional profile as Irish Moss, containing iodine, vitamins, minerals, and polysaccharides. It's valued for its potential health benefits, including supporting thyroid function, boosting immune health, and promoting digestion.

How to Prepare: Irish Sea Moss is prepared in the same way as Irish Moss, by soaking it in water to rehydrate and soften it before use. It can be used in culinary applications or consumed as a dietary supplement.

Dosage: The dosage of Irish Sea Moss depends on the form and intended use. As a dietary supplement, it's important to follow the recommended dosage on the product label or consult with a healthcare professional for personalized guidance.

How to Use: Irish Sea Moss can be used in various culinary applications, including soups, smoothies, desserts, and sauces. It can also be consumed as a dietary supplement in the form of capsules, powders, or extracts.

Side Effects: Similar to Irish Moss, Irish Sea Moss is generally considered safe for most people when consumed in moderate amounts. However, individuals with seaweed allergies or sensitivities to carrageenan should exercise caution. It's important to discontinue use if any adverse effects occur and to consult with a healthcare professional if you have any concerns.

Lymphalin:

Definition: Lymphalin is a herbal supplement formulated to support lymphatic system health. The lymphatic system plays a crucial role in immune function and waste removal in the body, and Lymphalin is designed to promote its proper function.

Ingredients: Lymphalin typically contains a blend of herbs and botanical extracts known for their traditional use in supporting lymphatic system health. Common ingredients may include cleavers, red clover, echinacea, burdock root, and calendula, among others.

How to Prepare: Lymphalin is usually available in capsule or liquid form. Capsules are taken orally with water, while liquid forms may be mixed with water or juice before consumption. It's important to follow the recommended dosage on the product label.

Dosage: The appropriate dosage of Lymphalin can vary depending on the specific product and individual needs. It's important to follow the recommended dosage on the product label or consult with a healthcare professional for personalized guidance.

How to Use: Lymphalin capsules are typically taken orally with water, while liquid forms may be mixed with water or juice before consumption. It's often recommended to take Lymphalin on an empty stomach for optimal absorption.

Side Effects: Lymphalin is generally considered safe for most people when used as directed. However, some individuals may experience mild side effects such as gastrointestinal discomfort or allergic reactions to certain ingredients. It's important to consult with a healthcare provider before starting any new supplement regimen, especially if you have underlying health conditions or are taking medications.

Manjakani:

Definition: Manjakani, also known as Quercus infectoria or oak gall, is a natural substance derived from the oak tree. It has been used for centuries in traditional medicine for its potential health benefits, particularly for women's health and vaginal tightening.

Ingredients: Manjakani contains various bioactive compounds, including tannins, flavonoids, and gallic acid. These compounds are believed to contribute to the herb's medicinal properties, including its potential as an astringent and antiseptic agent.

How to Prepare: Manjakani is typically available in powder, capsule, or liquid extract form. It can be taken orally or used topically depending on the intended use. For vaginal tightening, manjakani may be applied topically as a gel or inserted into the vagina in capsule form.

Dosage: The appropriate dosage of manjakani can vary depending on factors such as age, health status, and the specific preparation being used. It's important to follow the recommended dosage on the product label or consult with a qualified herbalist or healthcare professional for personalized guidance.

How to Use: Manjakani can be taken orally or used topically depending on the intended use. It's important to use manjakani products as directed and to discontinue use if any adverse effects occur.

Side Effects: Manjakani is generally considered safe for most people when used in moderate amounts. However, some individuals may experience allergic reactions or skin irritation when used topically. It's important to use manjakani under the guidance of a healthcare professional and to discontinue use if any adverse effects occur.

Bromide Plus Powder:

Definition: Bromide Plus Powder is a dietary supplement formulated to support thyroid health and promote overall well-being. It typically contains a blend of herbs and minerals that are believed to have beneficial effects on thyroid function.

Ingredients: Bromide Plus Powder often contains a combination of herbs such as bladderwrack, sea moss, and burdock root, along with minerals like iodine and potassium phosphate. These ingredients are thought to support thyroid function and maintain optimal iodine levels in the body.

How to Prepare: Bromide Plus Powder is usually mixed with water or juice to create a drinkable solution. It's important to follow the instructions on the product label for dosage and preparation.

Dosage: The dosage of Bromide Plus Powder can vary depending on the specific product and individual needs. It's crucial to consult with a healthcare professional or follow the recommended dosage on the product label to avoid potential side effects.

How to Use: Bromide Plus Powder is typically taken orally by mixing the recommended dosage with water or juice. It's important to shake or stir the mixture well before consuming it to ensure even distribution of the ingredients.

Side Effects: While Bromide Plus Powder is generally considered safe when used as directed, some individuals may experience side effects such as digestive discomfort or allergic reactions to certain ingredients. It's essential to consult with a healthcare provider before starting any new supplement regimen, especially if you have underlying health conditions or are taking medications.

Bugleweed:

Definition: Bugleweed, also known as Lycopusvirginicus, is a perennial herb native to North America and Europe. It has been used in traditional medicine to treat various conditions, including hyperthyroidism, anxiety, and insomnia.

Ingredients: Bugleweed contains several active compounds, including lithospermic acid, phenolic acids, and flavonoids. These compounds are believed to contribute to the herb's medicinal properties, particularly its ability to regulate thyroid function.

How to Prepare: Bugleweed is commonly consumed as a tea or tincture. To make tea, dried bugleweed leaves and flowers are steeped in hot water for several minutes before being strained and consumed. Tinctures are prepared by steeping the herb in alcohol or vinegar to extract its active compounds.

Dosage: The appropriate dosage of bugleweed can vary depending on factors such as age, health status, and the specific preparation being used. It's important to follow the recommended dosage on the product label or consult with a qualified herbalist or healthcare professional for personalized guidance.

How to Use: Bugleweed tea or tincture is typically taken orally. It can be consumed on its own or mixed with honey or other herbal teas for added flavor.

Side Effects: While bugleweed is generally considered safe for most people when used in moderation, excessive intake may cause digestive upset or allergic reactions in some individuals. Pregnant or breastfeeding women should avoid bugleweed due to its potential to stimulate uterine contractions. As with any herbal remedy, it's important to consult with a healthcare provider before using bugleweed, especially if you have underlying health conditions or are taking medications.

Burdock:

Definition: Burdock, scientifically known as Arctium lappa, is a biennial plant native to Europe and Asia but now found worldwide. It's part of the Asteraceae family and has been used for centuries in traditional medicine and culinary practices.

Ingredients: Burdock contains various nutrients, including carbohydrates, fiber, vitamins (such as vitamin B6, folate, and vitamin C), and minerals (including potassium, magnesium, and manganese). It also contains active compounds such as polyphenols and volatile oils.

How to Prepare: Burdock can be prepared and consumed in various ways. The roots, leaves, and seeds are all utilized for different purposes. The root is commonly used in cooking, herbal teas, tinctures, and supplements, while the leaves and seeds are sometimes used in herbal preparations.

Dosage: The appropriate dosage of burdock root can vary depending on the specific form and intended use. For culinary purposes, there are no strict dosage guidelines, but for supplements or herbal remedies, it's essential to follow the recommended dosage on the product label or consult with a healthcare professional.

How to Use: Burdock root can be used in cooking by peeling, slicing, and adding it to soups, stews, stir-fries, or salads. It can also be brewed into a tea or used to make tinctures or extracts for medicinal purposes. Some people may also take burdock root supplements in capsule or powder form.

Side Effects: While burdock is generally considered safe for most people when consumed in moderate amounts, some individuals may experience allergic reactions or digestive upset. Additionally, burdock may interact with certain medications or have adverse effects in individuals with certain health conditions, such as diabetes or allergies to plants in the Asteraceae family. It's important to consult with a healthcare provider before using burdock, especially if you have underlying health conditions or are taking medications.

THE END

www.ingramcontent.com/pod-product-compliance
Lightning Source LLC
Chambersburg PA
CBHW081555250726
48653CB00009B/3445